EKG Interpretation

Julie Johnson   RN, MSN

EKG Interpretation

ISBN-13: 978-1500736286

ISBN-10: 1500736287

Printed in the United States of America.

Dedication

To all who need a quick run-down on EKG Interpretation

The Conduction system of the heart

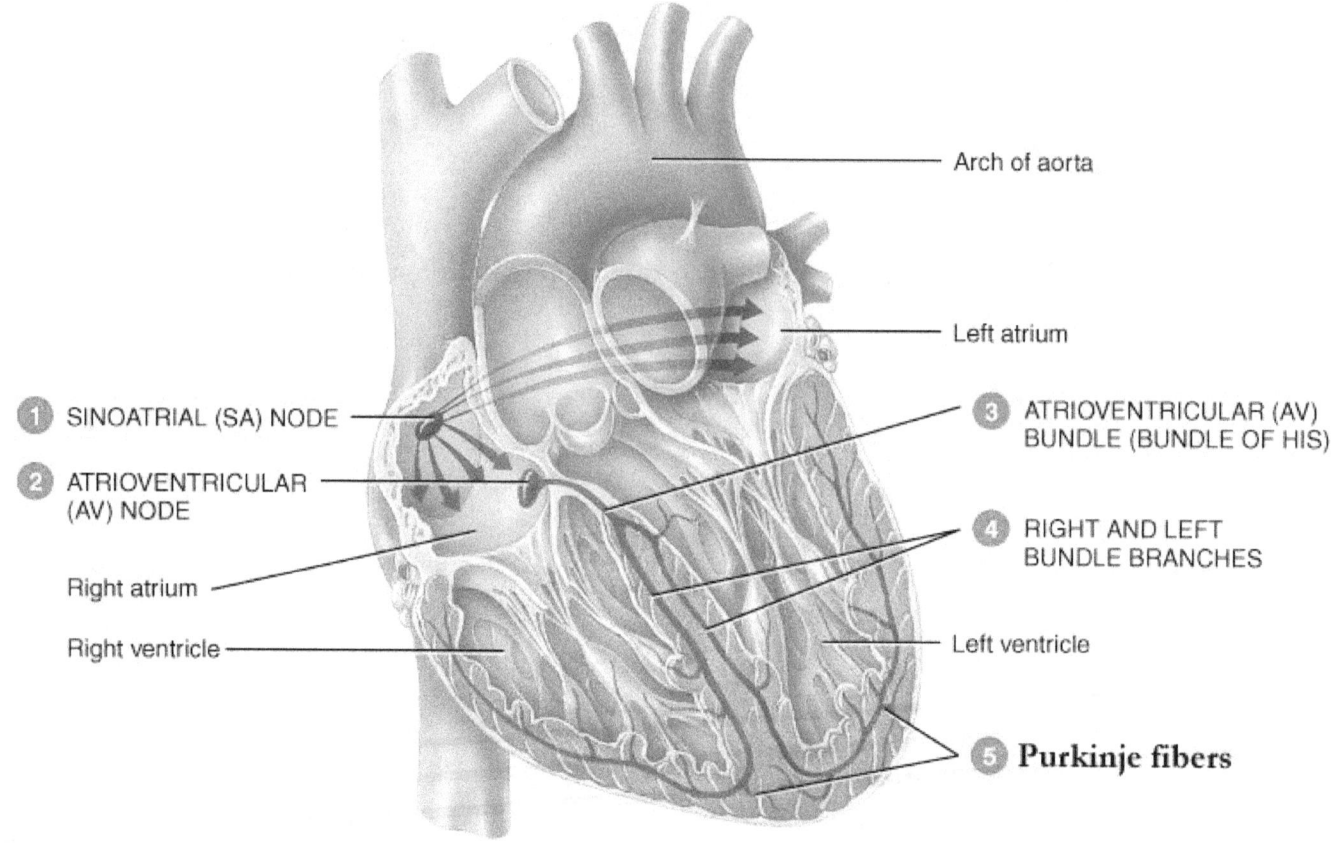

SINOATRIAL (SA) NODE

ATRIOVENTRICULAR (AV) NODE

Right atrium

Right ventricle

Arch of aorta

Left atrium

ATRIOVENTRICULAR (AV) BUNDLE (BUNDLE OF HIS)

RIGHT AND LEFT BUNDLE BRANCHES

Left ventricle

Purkinje fibers

Anterior view of frontal section

According to Baltazar (2009, p. 1), the heart consists of an electrical conduction system. The electrical conduction system consists of sinoatrial (SA) node, atrioventricular node, AV bundle, the bundle Branches (right and left), and purkinje fibres.

See this YouTube video http://www.youtube.com/watch?v=te_SY3MeWys

SA Node

Found in the upper posterior portion of the right atrial wall just below the opening of the superior vena cava. It is the primary pacemaker of the heart and has a normal firing rate of 60-100 beats per minute.

Internodal pathways

Consists of anterior, middle and posterior divisions that distribute electrical impulse generated by the SA node throughout the right and left atria to the atrioventricular (AV) node.

AV Junction:

AV node

Located at the posterior septal wall of the right atrium just above the tricuspid valve. There is a 1/10th of a second delay of electrical activity at this level to allow blood to flow from the atria to the ventricles.

Bundle of His

Found at the superior portion of the interventricular septum, it is the pathway that leads out of the SA node. It has an ability to initiate electrical impulses with an intrinsic firing rate of 40-60 beats per minute.

Bundle branches

Located at the interventricular septum, the bundle of His divides into the right and left bundle branches, the function of which is to conduct the electrical impulse to the Purkinje fibers.

Purkinje fibers

Found within the ventricular endocardium, it consists of a network of small conduction fibers that delivers the electrical impulses to the ventricular myocardium. This network has the ability to initiate electrical impulses and act as a pacemaker if the higher level pacemakers fail. The intrinsic firing rate is 20-40 beats per minute.

Sinoatrial (SA) node sets the pace for the heart naturally, by releasing regular electrical impulses. It is located at the upper right section of the right atrium. Sinoatrial node initiates electrical impulse that causes every single heartbeat. The impulses are transmitted via the atria causing the contraction of the cardiac muscles in a rhythmic wave. The pace rate of the SA node are based on individual needs of the human body.

The impulse initiated by the sinoatrial node is received by the atrioventricular(AV) node. Atrioventricular(AV) node is located in the lower side and to the middle of the right atrium. The Atrioventricular node similarly transmits the impulse through the ventricular nerve network. The result is contractions by the ventricles that resemble waves. The network of electrical fibers or nerves in the ventricles exits the antrioventricular node either on the right or left bundle branches. Simply said, there is something called the common bundle or atrioventricular bundle. The bundle branches into the right and left bundle branches with the left bundle going into the left ventricle and the right bundle going into the right ventricular. Impulse received through these nerve fibers result in the ventricular contractions.

Dubin (2000, p. 6) adds that, the heart being made up of up to a billion cells, consists of majority present in ventricular walls because of the amount of energy required to pump blood from the ventricles. Sinoatrial node rests when atrioventricular node is sending out impulse hence the heart does not stop for sinoatrial node to trigger another impulse. Therefore, there are two main stages: Depolarization(contraction) and Repolarization(Relaxation) of both the Atria and the ventricles.

Depolarization and Repolarization

Resting cardiac cells are negatively charged inside. When a cardiac cell is stimulated, sodium ions rush into the cell and potassium leaks out, changing into positivethe charge within. This electrical event is called depolarization and is expected to result in contraction. Depolarization flows from the endocardium to the myocardium to the epicardium.

During cell recovery, ions shift back to their original places and the cell recovers the negative charge inside. This is repolarization, and proceeds from the epicardium towards the endocardium. It results in myocardial relaxation.

1. Fundamentals of electrocardiogram

Dubin (2000, p. 6) notes that, electrocardiogram is a machine that records information on the heart's electrical activity. Electrodes connecting the electrocardiogram machine and the patient's heart can provide a means of recording electrical activity for analysis. The EKG machine main objective is to detect the flow of the patient's heart electrical activity by measuring on the patient's skin.

The functions of an electrocardiogram include computing a person's heart rate on the monitor, the duration of depolarization, repolarization and the length of time it takes to conduct the impulses. The electrocardiogram assesses the pacemaker's motions and regularity. When the patient is being administered medications, the electrocardiogram can be used to evaluate the extent of response of the body or heart to the medication. An electrocardiogram machine can give baseline reading of the heart prior, during and following a treatment or medical procedure.

An EKG machine generates information useful for the cardiologist or physician that is specific and resourceful. The information may include details of the heart's orientation in the chest. Additionally, the effects of fluid and electrolyte imbalance can be detected on the EKG machine. Features such as damages of blood vessels or ischemic cardiac muscles can be viewed and the mass shown for easy assessment.

The electrocardiogram is limited and may not show enough data on myocardium. When conducting the procedure the blood pressure as well as pulse is evaluated to support evidence on mechanical activity of the heart.

2. The electrocardiographic grid and waves

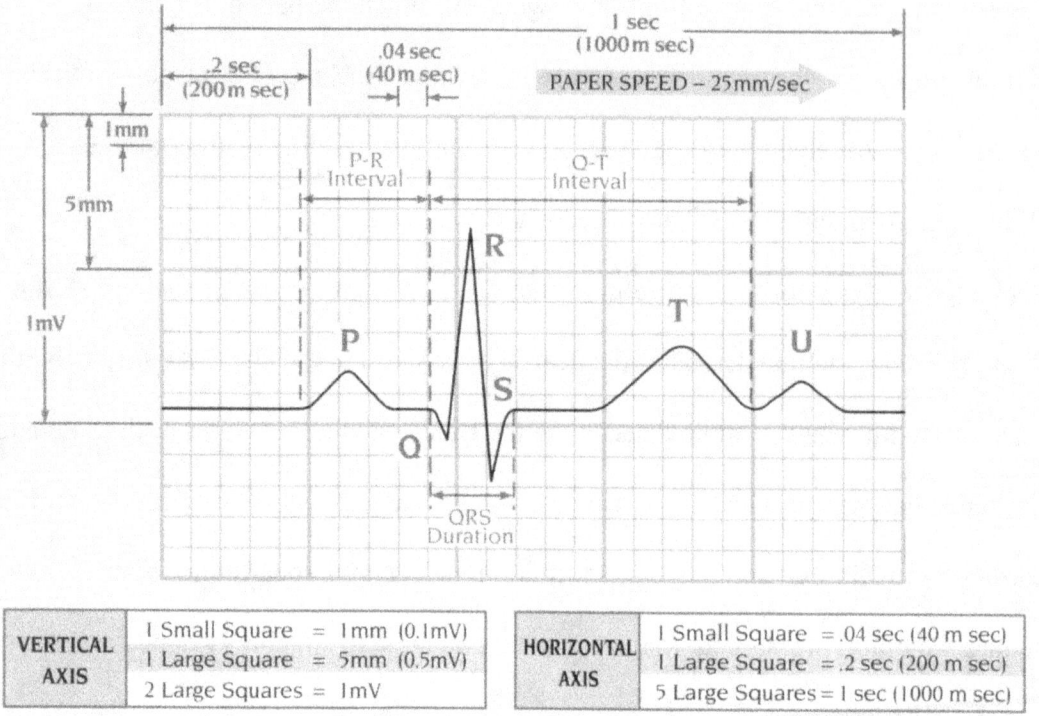

VERTICAL AXIS	1 Small Square = 1mm (0.1mV)
	1 Large Square = 5mm (0.5mV)
	2 Large Squares = 1mV

HORIZONTAL AXIS	1 Small Square = .04 sec (40 m sec)
	1 Large Square = .2 sec (200 m sec)
	5 Large Squares = 1 sec (1000 m sec)

The electrocardiographic grid is a representation of measurement of voltage plotted on a vertical axis. The axis is on time. The voltage and time are detected when electrodes that are connected to the machine provide a difference. Usually, a distance is deflected depending on the voltage to be measured.

The electrocardiogram waves are recorded on a specified graph designed for recording the waves. The graph is constructed in a manner that grid like square boxes of one millimeter squared appear. The electrocardiogram machine records twenty five millimeters per second. Consequently, one millimeter on the horizontal is equal to 0.04 seconds to 0.2 seconds intervals. On the vertical grid the electrocardiogram takes the measurement of the height on the graph which is tantamount to 10 millimeter of the standard calibration.

Estimation of the rate can be achieved through a countdown using the grid. On the grid small and large boxes on the grid can be counted between the two P waves that follow and the two R waves that follow. For the small boxes the number between two following P waves for atrial together with the number of squares between of two following R waves for ventricles rates are used. There are other methods to determine the heart rate like the R-R interval, 60-seconds times 10 interval, etc

See these videos on YouTube:

1. http://www.youtube.com/watch?v=S135w2_aDpo

2. http://www.youtube.com/watch?v=JNLdQRULhOo

3. http://www.youtube.com/watch?v=OAdMz9Wbn5E

3. Definition of waves, segments, intervals and junctions

Waves in an electrocardiogram are in the form of P, T or QRS waves. P waves denote atria depolarization. QRS waves stand for ventricle depolarization and T represents repolarization of the ventricle. Atria repolarization is almost impossible to be detected or viewed and when detected it is denoted as T wave. There are other waves that can appear abnormally such as delta waves. Delta waves slight portion of the QRS wave. Epsilon wave is seen towards the end of QRS wave. Osborn wave is also visible when QRS wave is ending in rigorous hypothermia (Canover 2003p. 41).

Wagner (2007, p. 11) notes that, a segment can be defined as the space between two waves. The PR segment begins after P wave and ends at the beginning of QRS complex. ST segments begin on end of QRS and ends at the beginning of T wave. In the cardiogram, a segment can also be described as isoelectric interval.

An interval can be defined as the region in a cardiogram that covers one segment with one or several waves. PR interval begins at beginning of the P wave and diminishes at the beginning of QRS. The difference between a PR interval and a PR segment is that a PR interval begins at the beginning of the P wave to the beginning of the Q wave, while a PR segment begins at the end of the P wave to the beginning of the Q wave. Some have questioned why it is not called the PQ interval, but NO, it is the PR interval. An interval can be interpreted as an impulse conducted from a section of atrium on the top towards the ventricle. QT interval begins where QRS starts and ends at the completion of T wave. An interval stands for the electrical systolic action performed by the heart. A junction is placed between a QRS and ST segment .

Simply put:

Waveform: refers to movement away from the isoelectric line with either upward (positive) deflection or downward (negative) deflection.

Segment: line between two waveforms.

Interval: waveform plus a segment.

Complex: several waveforms

4. The normal electrocardiograph waves and complexes

Normal electrocardiogram starts with a P wave that deflects atria depolarization (from right side to left then to inferiority) An active atrial depolarization appears on electrocardiogram as a P wave vertically in leads. The first precordial lead denoted as V1 is negative and signifies depolarization of posterity on the left side of the atrium. P wave amplitude does not exceed 2.5 millimeters and tenth of a second which is representative of a reduced amount of three boxes. Sometimes the P wave has a notch which separating left from right atrial actions. **P wave**: is the first deflection after the diastole, produced by atrial depolarization.

It is a smooth, round, not more than 2.5 mm high and no more than 0.11 sec

Positive in I,II, and V2 to V6. The normal P wave in standard, limb, and precordial leads does not exceed 0.11s in duration or 2.5mm in height. There is **no wave for atrial repolarization**, because is obscured by the larger QRS complex

PR segment detects isoelectric segment, which is deflected as well depolarized by abnormalities of atria caused by pericarditis or infarction of atrium. Normal PR measurements for the intervals are between 0.12 and 0.2 seconds.

QRS complexes timing is between 0.06 to 0.10 seconds. Q waves normally remains bellows 0.03 seconds and bellow 3milimetres depth. R wave remains within 20 to 25 millimeters height. QRS complex may be 30 to 105 degrees from the frontal axis indicating that there is a positive in the leads for the complexes. T wave faces identical direction with the QRS. The QT interval rate is subject to heart rate with the average normal heart beat being 70 beats per minute (Josephson, 2001, p. 57).

QRS complex Represents ventricular depolarization (activation). The ventricle is depolarized from the endocardium to the myocardium, to the epicardium. Normal duration is no more than 0.1 sec (otherwise stated as "less than .12 sec").

Q (q) wave: the initial negative deflection produced by ventricular depolarization.

R (r) wave: the first positive deflection produced by ventricular depolarization.

S (s) wave: the first negative deflection produced by the ventricular depolarization that follows the first positive deflection, (R) wave.

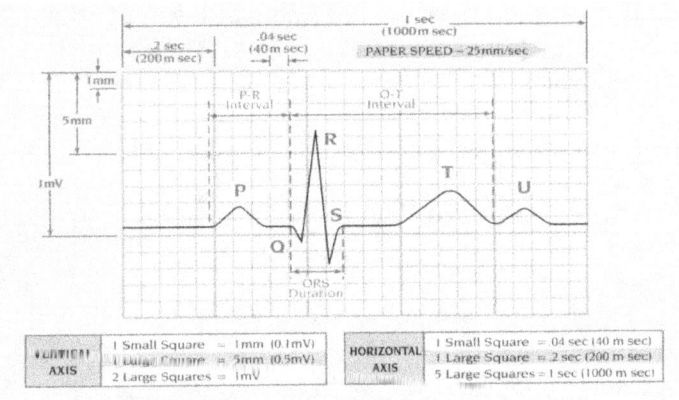

Ventricular Repolarization:

a. T wave: The first wave after the QRS complex has the following characteristics

The deflection produced by ventricular repolarization.

It is slightly asymmetric

No more than 5 mm in height

b. U wave: Is the deflection seen following the T wave but preceding the diastole.

Represents repolarization of Purkinje fibers

Round and symmetric less than 1.5 mm in height

A prominent U wave is due to hypokalemia (low potassium, blood level).

5. **The normal EKG segments, intervals and Junctions**

   a. PR segment this segment is measured from the end of the P wave to the beginning of the QRS complex. Represents depolarization of AV node and its delay and depolarization of the Bundle of His and the Bundle Branches.

   b. ST segment This segment represents the time of ventricular contraction and the beginning of repolarization of both ventricles. It is measured from end of QRS to the beginning of the T wave. The point where QRS complex and the ST segment meet is called "the junction" or "J point". ST segment is the most sensitive part of EKG changed by cardiac ischemia.

a. **PR Interval** Is defined as P wave plus PR segment and is measured from the beginning of P wave to the beginning of QRS complex. The normal interval is 0.12 – 0.2 sec.

b. **QT Interval** It represents the total ventricular activity (ventricular depolarization PLUS ventricular repolarization), and it is measured from the beginning of QRS to the end of T wave. The normal duration of this interval depends on the age and the HR.

c. **RR Interval.** It is important to determine the HR and its regularity..

RR interval: this is the interval between two R waves.

d. **J (RST) junction:** point at which QRS complex ends and ST segment begins.

e. **ST segment:** from J point to the onset of the T wave. This segment is compared to the PR segment to help identify myocardial ischemia or injury.

6. Analyzing the EKG strip

There are five steps that can be used for strip interpretation. The kind of rhythm determines the course of treatment to be administered. In the first stage, the electrocardiogram technician checks the rhythm to asses if the rhythm is normal or irregular. They assess if the rate is very fast, medium speed or too slow. 60 to 100 beats are considered the most appropriate hemodynamic hemorrhage. When the rate is below 60 beats or exceeds 100 beats, hemodynamic instability can be experienced.

The second stage is to evaluate if the heart rhythm is regular. The rhythms emanate from pace setters and are transmitted regularly. Irregular rhythm suggests that the beats are not released regularly and there could be abnormal beats which could be caused by certain conditions.

The third step involves examining all the components and the shape of waveforms. Check the measurement of the waves against the normal values like shape and duration.

The fourth step involves checking the position of the P wave. The electrocardiogram technologist finds out if P wave are present before the QRS complex, which denotes normal function of conduction from atria to ventricle. When p wave does not appear, the impulse could be emanating from a different part of the heart.

The final step establishes if all the complexes are alike. In a normal conduction each beat follow a similar pattern. Complexes that are diverse could indicate that impulses could be passing in wrong pathways.

See this YouTube video http://www.youtube.com/watch?v=WuKTkPJE-SE

Simply put:

A. ASSESS THE HEART RATE

1. **6 second Method**: The number of QRS complexes between 6 sec marks on the EKG paper is multiplied by 10. Used generally for estimating slow or irregular rhythms.

2. **Large Boxes Method**: count the number of large boxes between two consecutive RR (one RR interval) and divide into 300 for the ventricular rate; and count large boxes between two consecutive P waves for the atrial rate. Used mainly in regular rhythms.

3. **Small Boxes**: One minute has 1500 small boxes (0.04 sec). Count the number of small boxes between an RR interval and divide into 1500. This method is more accurate and is used for *regular rhythms only.*

4. **Sequence Method**: Select the R that falls on a dark vertical line. Number the next consecutive dark line as 300, 150, 100, 75, 60, and 50. Note where the next R wave falls in relation to the dark lines. That is the heart rate.

B. ASSESS RHYTHM/ REGULARITY

The HR is considered regular if all the RR or PP intervals on the EKG leads are equal. If there are changes in their durations the rhythm is irregular.

C. Identify and examine the P waves: Identify the P waves, PP interval and measure the size of the P wave in different leads.

D. Assess intervals (PR, QRS, QT): Measure each of these intervals and determine if they are normal.

E. Evaluate ST segments and T waves. ST segment elevation or depression and/or T wave abnormalities can suggest the presence of myocardial ischemia or injury.

F. General Evaluation and Conclusion: Notify the doctor for any abnormality that you can find on the EKG strip.

EKG interpretation and Pathology Recordings

Cardiac arrhythmias are due to the following mechanisms:

Arrhythmias of sinus origin - where electrical flow follows the usual conduction pathway but is too fast, too slow, or irregular. Normal sinus rate is 60-100 beats per minute. If the rate goes beyond 100 per minute, it is called sinus tachycardia. If the rate goes below 60 per minute, it is referred to as sinus bradycardia. *Ectopic rhythms* - electrical impulses originate from somewhere else other than the sinus node. *Conduction blocks* - electrical impulses go down the usual pathway but encounter blocks and delays. *Pre-excitation syndromes* - the electrical impulses bypass the normal pathway and, instead, go down an accessory shortcut.

Randal (2004, p. 54) mentions that when interpreting electrocardiogram, it is important to identify the normal behavior of the heart, that is the baseline method. A heart in good condition will have a Normal Sinus Rhythm. Any deviation from a normal sinus rhythm is usually a thing of concern. Some deviations like sinus dysrhythmia are of low concern while rhythms like Ventricular fibrillation are life threatening emergencies. Let us take a look at some common EKG Strips.

Normal Sinus Rhythm

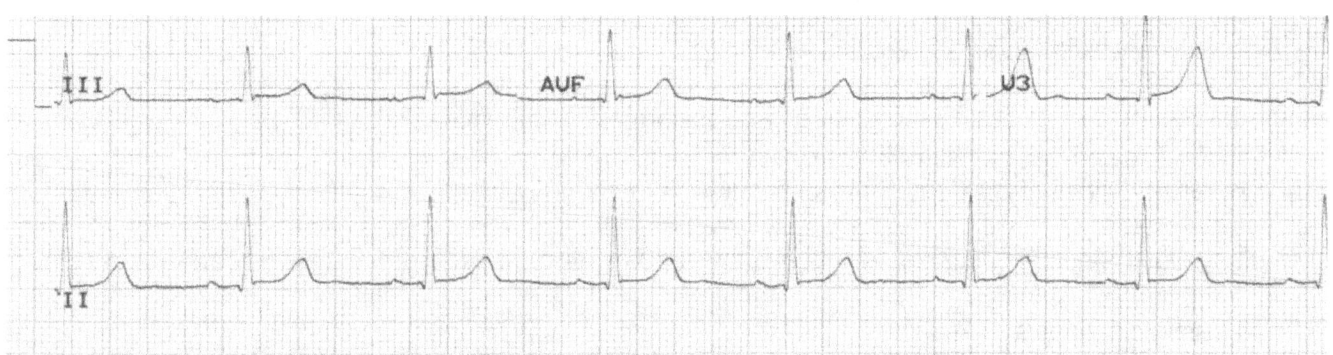

Originated from the SA Node and has the following characteristics:

a. Heart Rate of 60 – 100 bpm

b. Similar P waves in all the leads in front of all QRS complexes

c. A constant PR interval of 0.12 to 0.2 sec in all the leads,

d. Regular rhythm

e. QRS complex < 0.12

f. QT interval < 0.40

Sinus Bradycardia

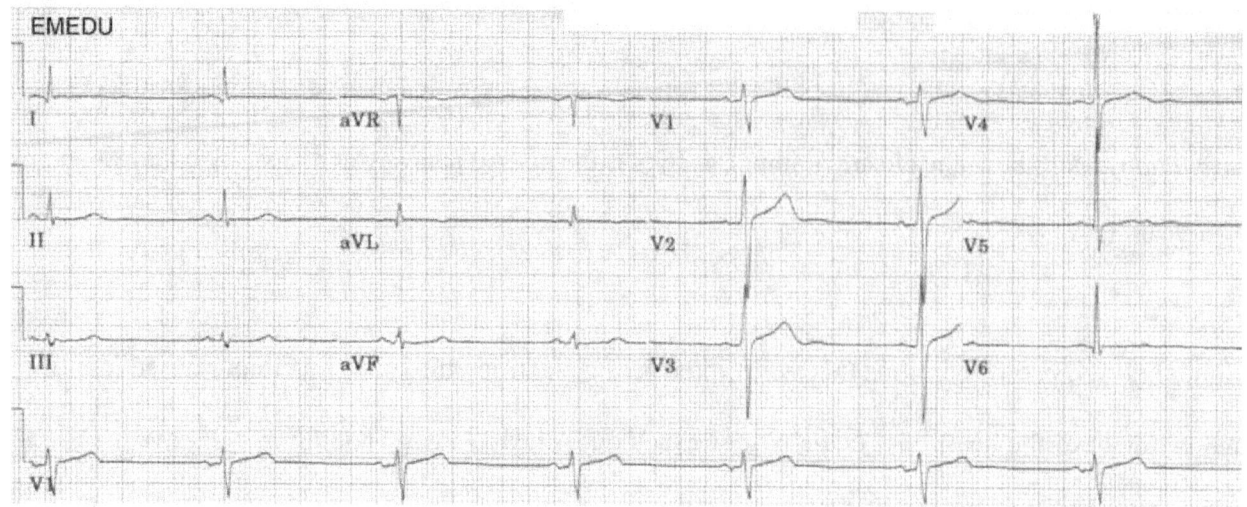

Bradycardia may be normal for athletes. It may also be normal in some individuals during sleep. Causes include vomiting, bearing down to have a bowel movement or diseases like myocardial infarction, obstructive jaundice and increased intracranial pressure. Medications such as digitalis, calcium-channel blockers and other anti-arrhythmic medications can also contribute to this rhythm. Features include:

a. HR less than 60 bpm

b. Normal equal P and QRS in all the leads, as well as normal PR intervals

c. . Bradycardia decreases the blood flow in the brain and other body tissues.

One can say that Sinus Bradycardia has the features of Normal Sinus Rhythm except a heart rate lower than 60 beats per minutes.

Sinus Tachycardia

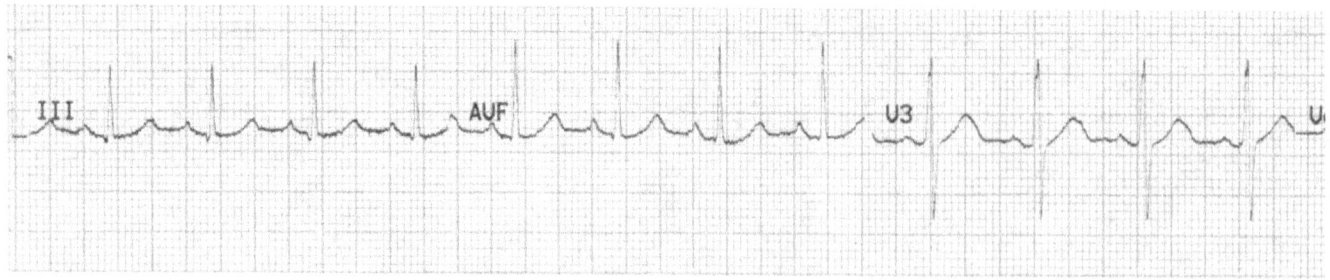

During stress and exercise, Sinus Tachycardia is normal. If Sinus Tachycardia persists at rest, conditions such as fever, dehydration, blood loss, anemia, anxiety, heart failure, hypermetabolic states and consumptions of stimulants such as cocaine, methamphetamine, etc may be the cause. Drugs that can cause Sinus Tachycardia include: atropine, isoproterenol, epinephrine, dopamine, dobutamine, norepinephrine, nitroprusside and caffeine. Sinus Tach increases the heart's need for oxygen. Treatment includes finding out the underlying cause and treating it. Drugs of choice include: digitalis, beta-blockers, calcium-channel blockers, sedatives and other antiarrhythmic medications. Features include:

a. HR: 100 - 150 bpm

b. Normal equal P and QRS in all the leads, as well as normal PR intervals (0.12-0.20sec)

c. PR interval: 0.12-0.20 sec

d. QRS: < 0.12

Rhythm: Regular.

Sinus Tach originates from the SA Node.

Supraventricular Tachycardia (Life threatening)

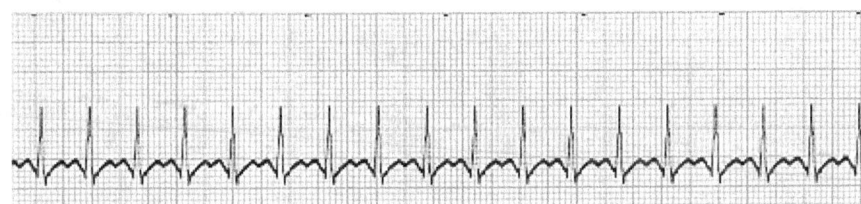

Atrial Tachycardia (AT) is caused by an irritable focus in the atria that fires electrical impulses after the normal firing of the SA node pacemaker. **HR is regular between 150 and 250 bpm.**

AV Reentry Tachycardia is caused when the electrical impulse passes through a passage other than AV node. Cardiac rhythm is regular but up to 250 bpm. P waves are often hidden by the QRS complexes or the QRS complexes that follow a P wave are different and with different PR interval (AV Nodal Reentry Tachycardia **AVNRT**).

In cases with **AV Reentry Tachycardia (AVRT) QRS** complexes are greater than 0.12 sec with a slurred up strike (delta wave) seen in one or more leads.

Atrial flutter

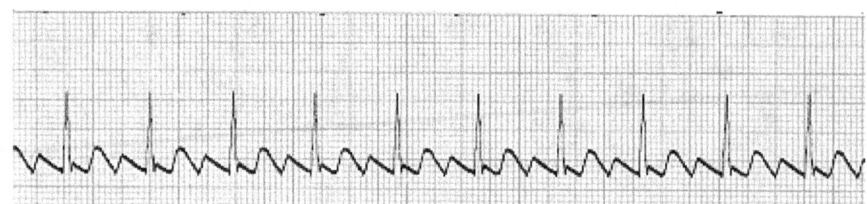

Atrial Flutter: Notice that there are no more "P" waves, instead a typical saw-tooth-like wave, called "F" wave is seen in the above recording. This rhythm leads to loss of atrial contraction resulting in decreased cardiac output 20-30%. Risks associated with this rhythm include: mural thrombi, hemodynamic instability, systemic or pulmonary embolism, etc. It is a life threatening situation. Cardioversion is usually done if it is an acute arrhythmia. If it is a chronic rhythm that is not responsive to medications, it is important that the patient be evaluated and possibly placed on an anticoagulant medication.

a. Atrial Flutter is characterized by rapid depolarization of a single atrial focus at a rate of 250-350 bpm.

b. Because the AV node cannot transmit every impulse at excessive rates, there is typically a slower ventricular rate (often appearing as a 2:1, 3:1, 4:1, etc. conduction ratio).

c. Typical **saw-toothed waves,** named "F" waves, followed by almost normal QRS complexes with a slower rate are seen in all the leads.

Atrial Fibrillation

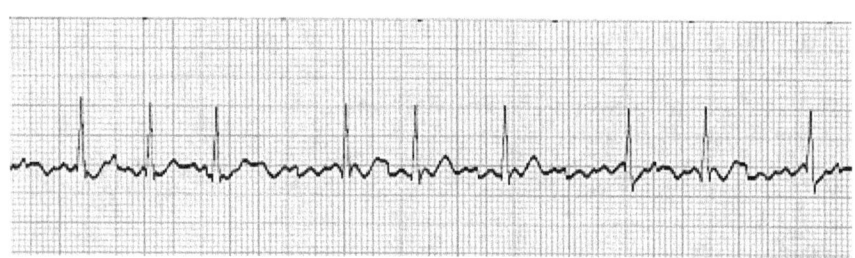

There are no "P" waves, instead they are substituted by small trembling waves, while QRST complex are almost normal and fired with a different rate.
Atrial fibrillation is caused by multiple irritable sites all over the atria firing at a rate exceeding 350 bpm.

These rapid impulses cause quivering (fibrillation) of the muscular fibers, which results in a drastic decrease in the cardiac output, blood stagnation and the formation of a clot. Cardiac output is reduced with the loss of "Atrial Kick" because the atria are not contracting. If the ventricular rate are also fast, there will be further decreased cardiac output. The patient is at risk of pulmonary embolism or stroke. Causes: MI, Rheumatic Heart

Disease, COPD, CHF, Ischemic Chest Trauma, CAD and open heart Surgery. Cardioversion is usually done in acute cases.

- No identifiable P waves can be seen, **_fibrillatory erratic "f" waves_** are seen in all the leads. Ventricular rhythm is very irregular, with a much slower rate than the atria. This is seen in all leads.

- Controlled atrial fibrillation: Average ventricular rate is less than 100 bpm.

- Uncontrolled atrial fibrillation: Average ventricular rate is over 100 bpm.

Premature Ventricular Complex

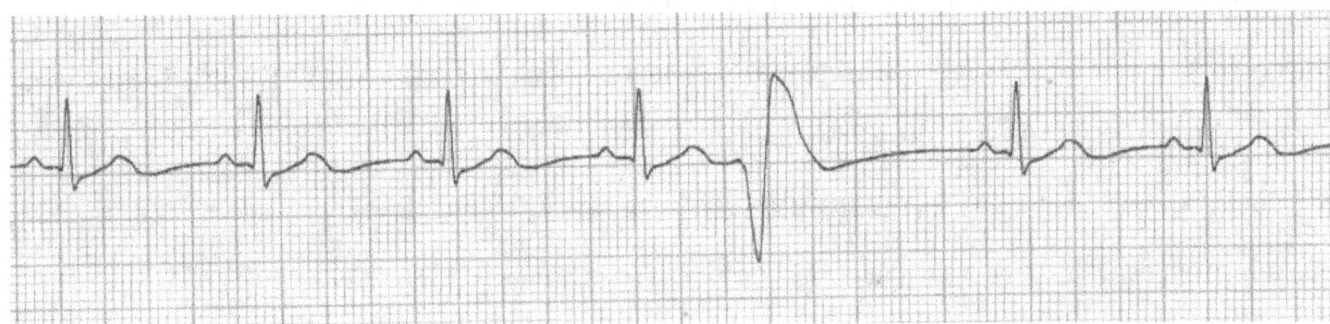

Notice the difference between the normal QRS complexes and the wide inverted abnormal QRS of the PVC and the full compensatory pause.

A premature ventricular complex arises from an irritable site within the ventricles. PVCs can appear as single, couplets, or triplets. Six or more PVCs occurring in a row are considered a run of V-Tach. PVC may appear in the same shape or in different shapes. When they appear in the same shape, they are believed to arise from a common point or focus, therefor are referred to as unifocal PVCs, but when they arise from different foci, they are referred to as multifocal PVCs.

The QRS of PVC is typically greater than 0.12 sec because the ventricular depolarization is abnormal or *aberrant*. The origin is usually ventricular/purkinje fibres. Causes: Increased catecholamines as seen in heightened emotions, stimulants such as coffee, nicotine, ethanol, cocaine, amphetamins, AMI, CHF, digitalis, increased vagal tones, hypoxia, acidosis, hypokalemia, hypomagnesemia, acidosis, ischemia, hypoxia and open heart surgery. T waves are usually in opposite direction of the QRS complex . A full compensatory pause usually follows a PVC. The rate and the PR interval are that of the underlying rhythm. The most important treatment is to find out and treat the underlying causes. Drugs of choice include beta blockers, procainamide, lidocaine, amiodarone, etc.

Ventricular Tachycardia

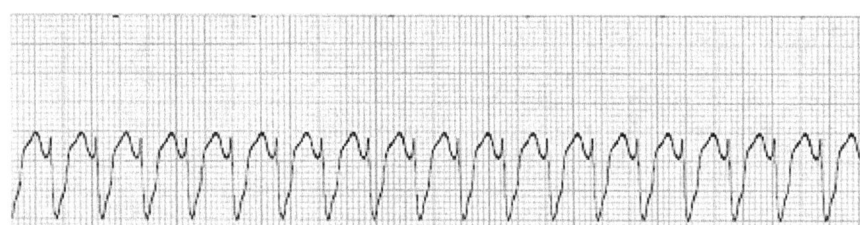

Ventricular Tachycardia (V-Tach) is characterized by 3 or more PVC's in a row at a rate over 100 bpm. If V-Tach occurs for more than 30 sec is called *sustained Ventricular Tachycardia*. The main characteristics of this rhythm are: Regular fast rhythm 100 to 250 bpm, No P waves or P waves may be present if SA node is functional, however, there is no relation to the QRS Wide, bizarre QRS complexes > 0.12 with T waves pointing in opposite direction from main QRS direction (T waves may be difficult to identify). If QRS complexes are different in size it is called *Polymorphic V-Tach* or "Torsades de Pointes".

Causes of V-Tach include hypoxia, acidosis, cardiomyopathy, mitral valve prolapse, digitalis toxicity, antiarrhythmics, electrolyte imbalance, liquid protein diets, increased intracranial pressure and central nervous system disorders. The longer a patient stays in V-Tach, the more difficult it is to convert to a normal rhythm. Stable patients may be medicated to attempt a chemical conversion. Unstable patients are treated promptly with defibrillation. **It is a life threatening emergency.**

Ventricular Fibrillation (Life threatening)

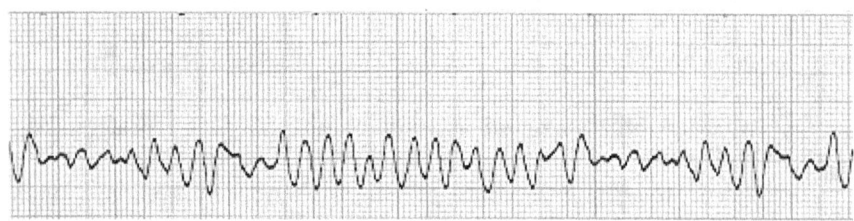

It is produced by multiple electrical sites firing electrical impulses at the same time resulting in quivering of the ventricles myocardial muscle fibers, but not a uniform contraction.

The rhythm is a chaotic deflection of different waves that vary in size, shape and duration.

There are no normal visible waves. There is no contraction, there is no blood ejected in the blood vessels, so the blood can clot. This is a medical emergency, which requires defibrillation and CPR.

Asystole (No electrical activity in the heart)

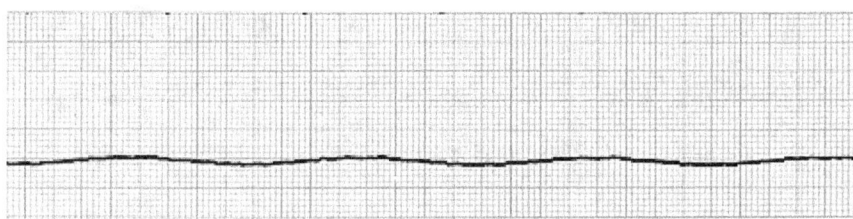

First Degree Heart Block, Type I

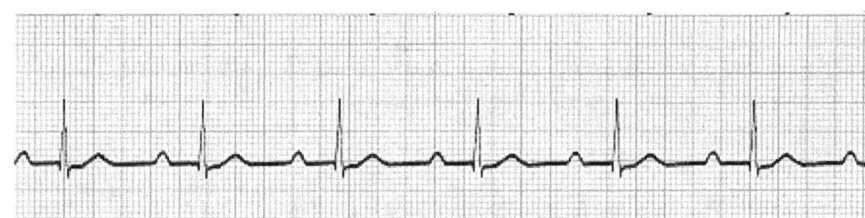

It is characterized by a delay of impulses at the level of AV node. . *PR interval is prolonged and is greater than 0.2 sec*

Second Degree Heart Block Type I

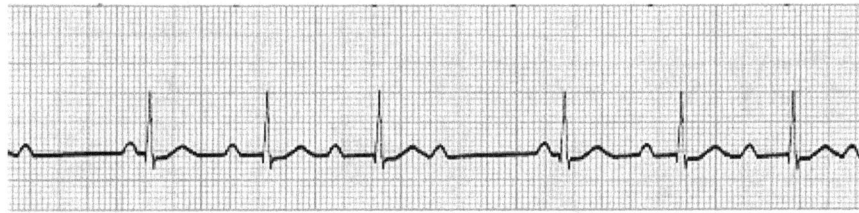

PR interval lengthens in each interval until one QRS disappears

Type II Second Degree AV Block (Mobitz II)
It is a more serious pathology.

Conducted P waves have a constant PR interval; but there are always non-conducted P waves between cardiac cycles, usually producing a "conduction ratio" between atria and ventricles (i.e. 2 P waves for each QRS, or 3 P waves for each QRS)

Third Degree AV Block. This type of AV block is also called a Complete Heart Block, or CHB, because impulses generated by the SA node are completely blocked before reaching the ventricular muscle fibers. The atria and ventricles beat independently from each other. Second degree blocks can progress in third degree blocks, especially after an inferior MI (myocardial Infarction). The third degree block's characteristics are:

-Atrial rate is greater than ventricular rate

-P waves are normal, there are no measurable PR intervals

-The atrial rhythm (P waves) is regular; AND the ventricular rhythm is regular (QRS complexes).

There is no relationship between P waves and QRS complexes

If the escape rhythm is junctional, the QRS complexes may appear normal in width and the ventricular rate may be slightly higher

If the escape rhythm is ventricular, the QRS complexes will be abnormally wide with a slower ventricular rate.

7. Artifacts of EKG Recording

Somatic Tremor

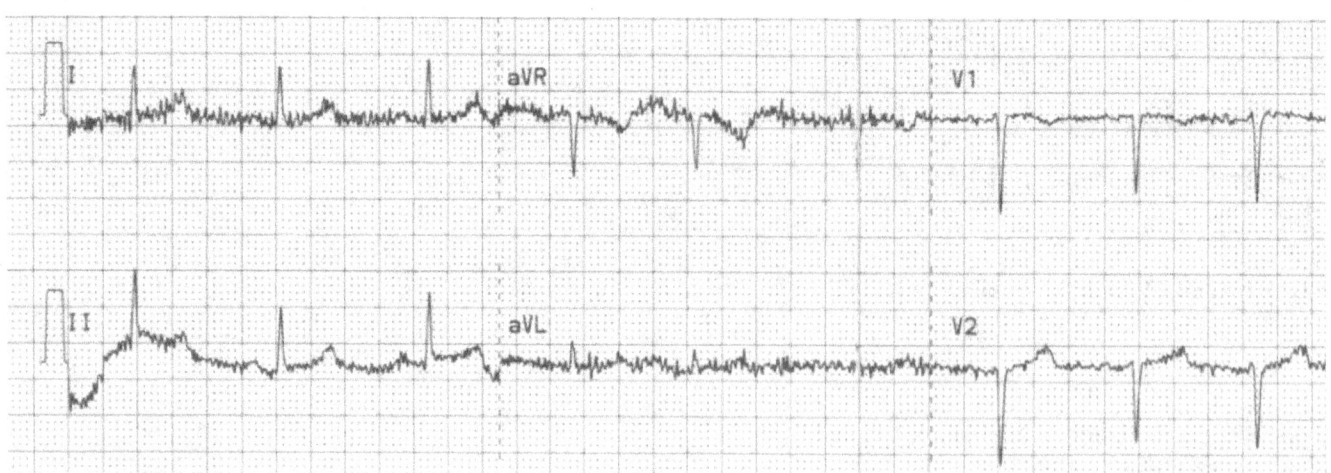

Wandering Baseline

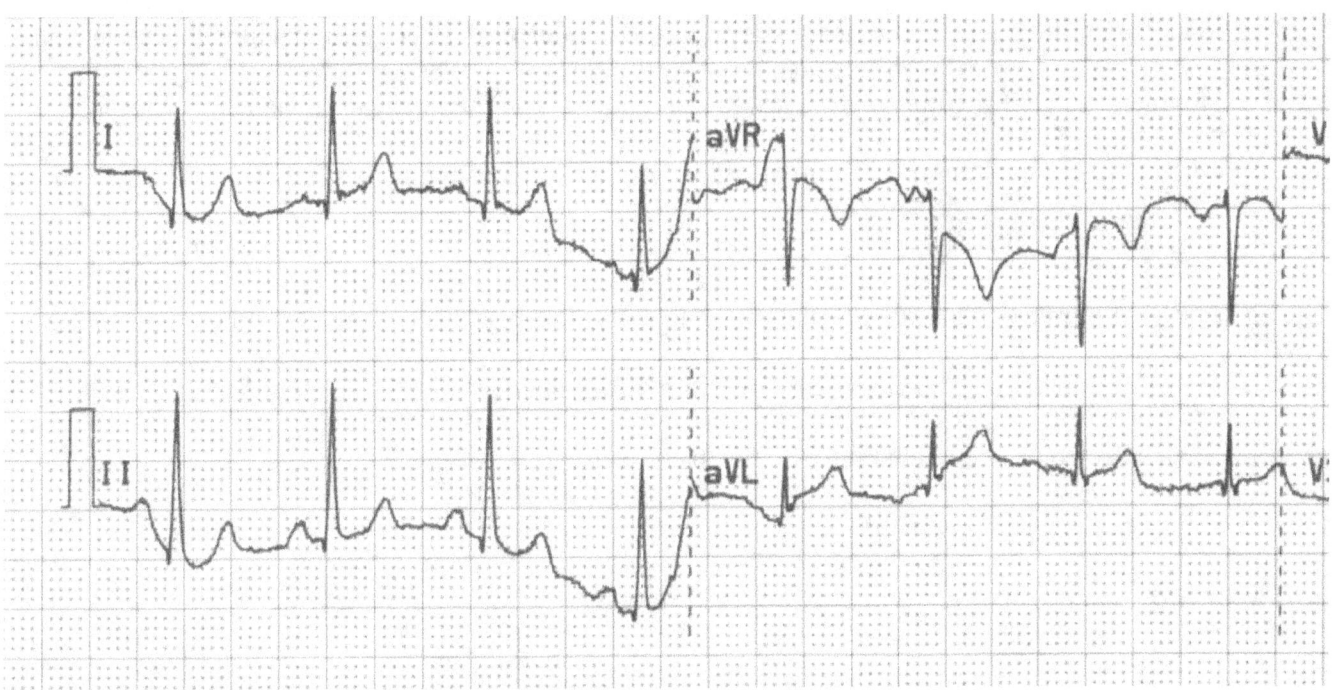

60 Cycle Circumference

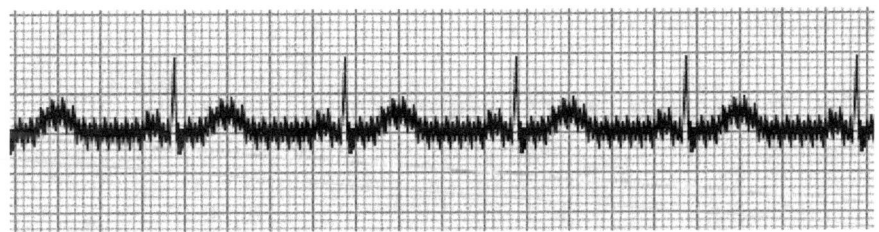

EKG AMBULATORY SYSTEMS: The following are the basic requirements for ambulatory systems. They include consumption of power that is low, detection for low voltage power battery, ability to obtain the electrocardiogram leads simultaneously. Wireless communication, small in size, operation time of the battery should be a minimum of 24 hours continuously and obtain a recording ability with functions of display and enough storage in real time.

It consists of two blocks which are fitted with a transmitter and a receiver. The transmitters function is to condition, process, digitalize, encode and transmit to the electrocardiogram leads together with battery information to be received. The receiver detects information transmitted via the electrocardiogram where it is decoded. The Signal is send computer for recording display and storage.

8. Conclusion

An electrocardiogram technologist assists in the use of electrocardiogram machine in a physician's room or laboratory to generate information used for diagnosis. The human heart is made up of muscle tissue, located between the lungs and pump blood to different parts of the body. The electrocardiogram records hearts activity and presents them on a screen or recorded tape where the information is analyzed. The electrocardiogram records heart orientation, heart disturbance, effects of medication on heart and base line reading of heart activity. The electrocardiogram requires interpretation from an expert. Some abnormalities detected can be treated for patients to recover.

References

Baltazar, R. F. (2009). *Basic and Bedside Electrocardiography.*New York: Lippincott Williams & Wilkins.

Canover, M. B. (2003) *Understanding Electrocardiography.* Philadelphia, PA: Mosby.

Dubin, D. (2000). *Rapid Interpretation of EKG's.* Florida, USA: Cover Publishing Company.

Ecman, M. (1990). *ECG interpretation.* New York: Springhouse Corporation.

Gomella, L. (2006). *Clinician's Pocket Reference.* New York: McGraw-Hill Medical.

Goldberger, A. L. (2012). *Clinical Electrocardiography: A Simplified Approach.* Philadelphia, PA: Saunders.

Hummel, J. D., Kalbfleisch, S. J. and J. M. Dillon. (1999). *Pocket Guide for Cardiac Electrophysiology.* Philadelphia: W. B. Saunders Company.

Josephson, M. E. (2001). *Clinical Cardiac Electrophysiology: Techniques and Interpretations.* Philadelphia: Lippincott Williams & Wilkins Publishers.

Randal, D. C. (2004). *ECG Interpretation.* Hayes Barton Press.

Wagner, G. S. (2007). *Marriott's Practical Electrocardiography*. New York: Lippincott   Williams &

Wilkins.

Common Cardiovascular Agents

One of the essentials of quality care of a patient who is having an acute myocardial infarction is pharmacological therapy. The following are the common pharmacological agents used.

Oxygen

Oxygen should be given to all patients with acute chest pain that may be due to cardiac ischemia, suspected hypoxemia of any cause, and cardiopulmonary arrest. Prompt treatment of the hypoxemia may prevent cardiac arrest. For patients breathing spontaneously, masks and nasal cannulas can be used to administer oxygen.

Epinephrine

Epinephrine is indicated in the management of cardiac arrest. The chance of successful defibrillation is enhanced by administration of epinephrine and proper oxygenation.

Isoproterenol (Isuprel)

Isoproterenol produces an overall increase in heart rate and myocardial contractility, but newer agents have replaced it in most clinical settings. It is contraindicated in the routine treatment of cardiac arrest.

Dopamine (Intropin)

Dopamine is indicated for significant hypotension in the absence of hypovolemia. Significant hypotension is present when systolic blood pressure is less than 90 mmHg with evidence of poor tissue perfusion, oliguria, or changes in mental status. It should be used at the lowest dose that produces adequate perfusion of vital organs.

Beta Blockers: Propranolol, Metoprolol, Atenolol, and Esmolol

Beta blockers reduce heart rate, blood pressure, myocardial contractility, and myocardial oxygen consumption which make them effective in the treatment of angina pectoris and hypertension.

They are also useful in preventing atrial fibrillation, atrial flutter, and paroxysmal supraventricular tachycardia. Adverse effects of beta blockers are hypotension, congestive heart failure and broncho-spasm.

Lidocaine

Lidocaine is the drug of choice for the suppression of ventricular ectopy, including ventricular tachycardia and ventricular flutter. Excessive doses can produce neurological changes, myocardial depression, and circulatory depression. Neurological toxicity is manifested as drowsiness, disorientation, decreased hearing ability, paresthesia, and muscle twitching, and

eventual seizures.

Verapamil

Verapamil is used in the treatment of paroxysmal supraventricular tachycardia (PSVT), effective

in terminating more than 90% of episodes of PVST in adults and infants. Verapamil is also useful in slowing ventricular response to atrial flutter and fibrillation. Vigilant monitoring of blood pressure is recommended due to hypotension that could occur.

Digitalis

Digitalis increases the force of cardiac contraction as well as cardiac output.. Digitalis toxicity is common with an incidence of up to 20%. Patients require constant monitoring for signs and symptoms of toxicity such as: yellow vision, nausea, vomiting, and drowsiness.

Morphine Sulfate

It is the traditional drug of choice for the pain and anxiety associated with acute myocardial infarction. In high doses, morphine sulfate may cause respiratory depression. It is a controlled substance and has a tendency for abuse and addiction.

Nitroglycerin

Nitroglycerin is a powerful smooth muscle relaxant effective in relieving angina pectoris. It is effective for both exertional and rest angina. Headache is a common consequence following the administration of this drug. Hypotension may occur and patients should be instructed to sit or lie down while taking nitroglycerin.

Review Questions

1) What is a normal sinus rate?
   a. 20-60 bpm
   b. 60-100 bpm
   c. 100-120 bpm
   d. 120-140 bpm

2) What is an arrhythmia of sinus origin?
   a. When electrical flow is disrupted and originates in the ventricles
   b. When the electrical flow is disrupted, but is still a normal heart rate
   c. When the electrical flow is stopped
   d. When the electrical flow is normal, but the heart rate is too fast or slow

3) What is an ectopic rhythm?
   a. When the electrical flow is normal, but the beat is irregular
   b. When the electrical flow is normal, but the heartbeat is too fast
   c. When the electrical flow originates from anywhere other than the sinus node
   d. None of the above

4) A heart rate with a normal electrical flow, but more than 100 BPM is called:
   a. Sinus tachycardia
   b. Ventricular fibrillation
   c. Sinus bradycardia
   d. Ventricular tachycardia

5) A heart rate with normal electrical flow, but fewer than 60 bpm is called:
   a. Sinus tachycardia
   b. Ventricular fibrillation
   c. Sinus bradycardia
   d. Ventricular tachycardia

6) What is a conduction block?
   a. The foundation for electrical impulse
   b. A type of brick used to build cardiac wards

    c. Blocks or delays along electrical pathways
    d. All of the above

7) What is a pre-excitation syndrome?
    a. Electrical impulses bypassing normal electrical pathways
    b. A type of sinus rhythm
    c. A block or delay among electrical pathways
    d. A type of tachycardia

8) The following is an example of

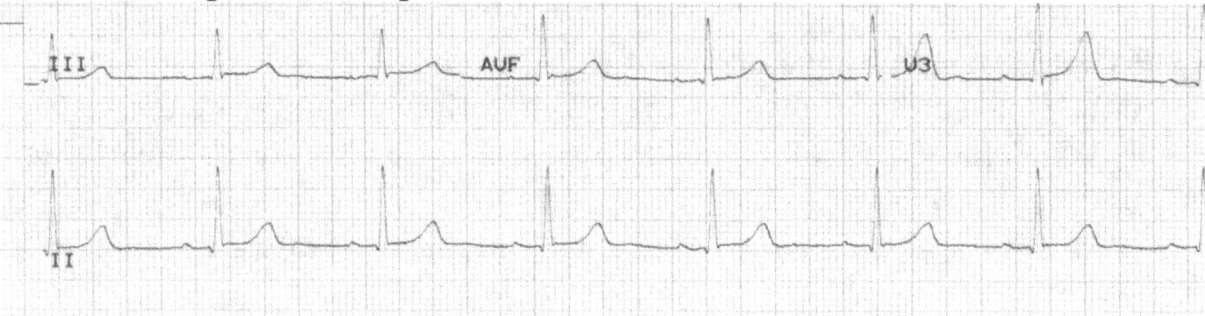

    a. Pre-excitation syndrome
    b. A block or delay
    c. A normal sinus rhythm
    d. Atrial fibrillation

9) Which of the following is not a part of a normal sinus rhythm?
    a. 60-100 BPM
    b. QRS complex < 0.12
    c. Regular rhythm
    d. Inverted P waves in the front of all QRS complexes

10)   Which of the following statements about bradycardia is false?
    a. It is a heart rate of less than 60 BPM
    b. It is characterized by normal equal P and QRS in all leads
    c. It shows the characteristics of normal sinus rhythms except the rate
    d. It is never normal in any person

11)   When is sinus tachycardia normal?
    a. When a person becomes elderly
    b. Never
    c. During stress and exercise

d. During rest

12)	The following is an example of

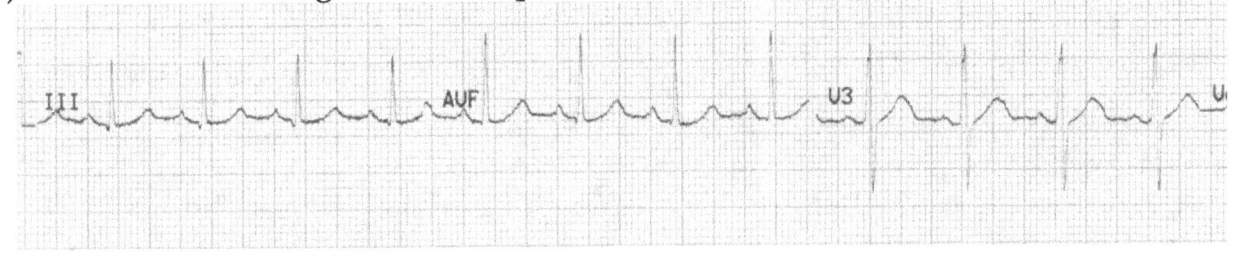

a. A normal sinus rhythm
b. Sinus tachycardia
c. Sinus Bradycardia
d. Supraventricular Tachycardia

13)	The following is an example of

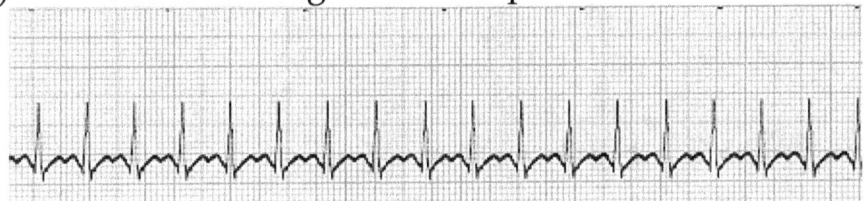

a. A normal sinus rhythm
b. Sinus tachycardia
c. Sinus bradycardia
d. Supraventricular Tachycardia

14)	A saw-tooth like wave called "F" wave that causes a 20%-30% decrease
in cardiac output is called:
a. Supraventricular Tachycardia
b. AV reentry Tachycardia
c. Atrial flutter
d. Atrial fibrillation

15)	Atrial fibrillation is characterized by:
a. Small trembling waves rather than "P" waves
b. Defined "P" waves, but no "S" waves
c. Small trembling waves rather than "T" waves
d. None of the above

16)	Which of the following is characterized by 3 or more PVC's in a row?
a. Atrial tachycardia

b. Ventricular tachycardia
c. Asystole
d. Premature ventricular complex

17)   Which of the following is produced because of multiple electrical sites firing at the same time, causing quivering?
a. Asystole
b. Ventricular fibrillation
c. Atrial fibrillation
d. Ventricular tachycardia

18)   When the PR interval is longer than 0.2 seconds it is:
a. First degree heart block, type I
b. Third degree heart block, type I
c. Second degree heart block, type III
d. Fourth degree heart block, type II

19)   A complete heart block is also known as:
a. A second degree AV block
b. A third degree aneurism
c. A first degree ventricular block
d. A third degree AV block

20)   Which of the following shows an inverted QRS with a full compensatory pause?
a. A second degree AV block
b. Asystole
c. A premature ventricular complex
d. Sinus bradycardia

21)   A normal sinus rhythm should have a QRS complex that is:
a. Less than 0.5
b. Less than 0.10
c. Less than 0.12
d. Greater than 0.12

22)   The following is an example of

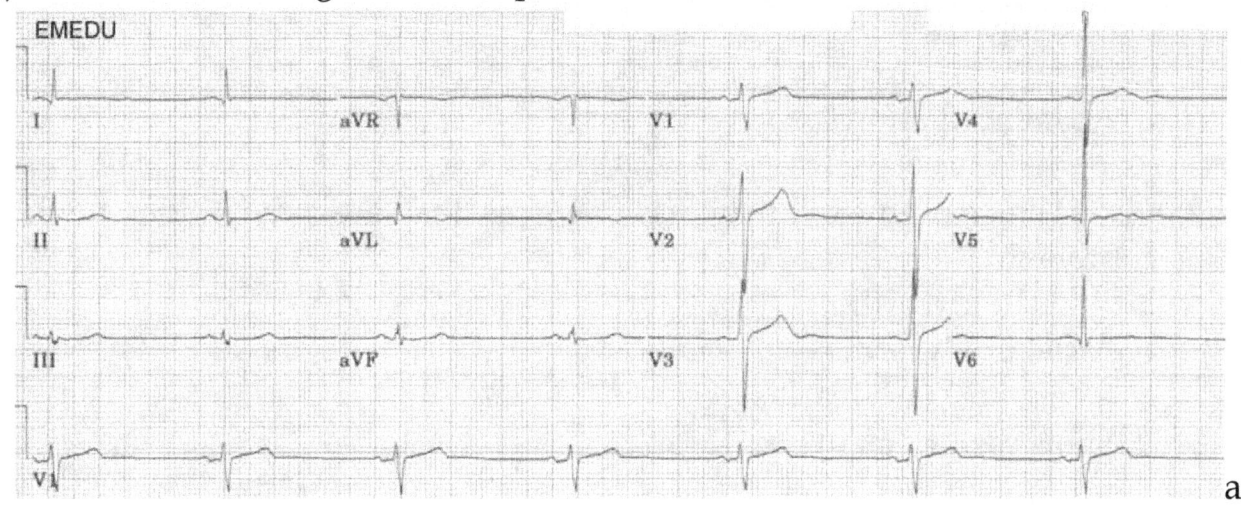

EMEDU

a

. Sinus tachycardia
b. Sinus bradycardia
c. Ventricular tachycardia
d. Ventricular bradycardia

23)   Which of the following causes sinus bradycardia?
  a. Obstructive jaundice
  b. Vomiting
  c. Increased intracranial pressure
  d. All of the above

24)   Which of the following causes sinus tachycardia?
  a. Exercise
  b. Caffeine
  c. Cardiac problems
  d. All of the above

25)   Which of the following statements about supraventricular tachycardia is false?
  a. The heart rate is between 150 and 250 BPM
  b. It is caused by an irritable focus in the atria
  c. It is not life threatening
  d. It is an irregular heartbeat

26)   Which of the following occurs when an electrical impulse passes through a passage other than the AV node and is characterized by a rhythm of up to 250 BPM?

a. AV reentry tachycardia
b. Asystole
c. Sinus tachycardia
d. Atrial fibrillation

27)   Which of the following has P waves that are often hidden by the QRS complex?
a. Sinus bradycardia
b. Atrial bradycardia
c. AV reentry tachycardia
d. Sinus reentry tachycardia

28)   The following is an example of

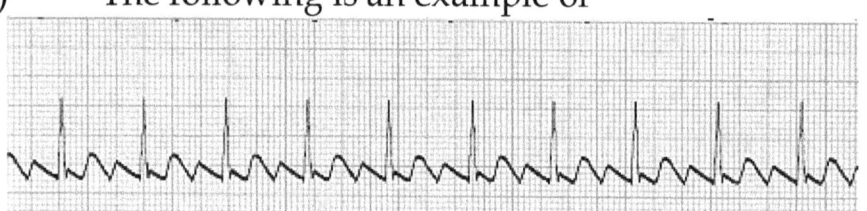

a. AV reentry bradycardia
b. Atrial flutter
c. Ventricular flutter
d. Asystole

29)   Which of the following could possible cause atrial flutter?
a. Pulmonary embolism
b. hemodynamic instability
c. Mural thrombi
d. All of the above

30)   The following is an example of

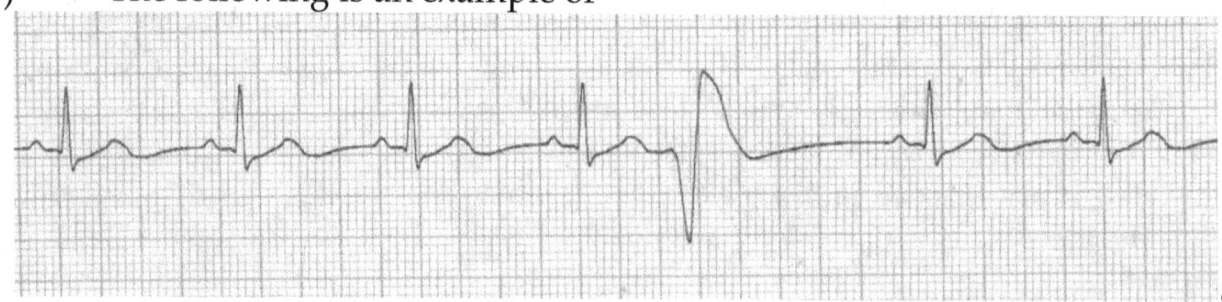

a. Atrial fibrillation
b. Premature ventricular complex
c. Sinoatrial complex

d. Sinoatrial delay

31)   Atrial fibrillation is caused by:
    a. Multiple irritable sites all over the atria firing at more than 350 BPM
    b. Multiple irritable sites all over the ventricle firing at more than 300 BPM
    c. Ventricular failure
    d. Atrial failure

32)   The following is an example of
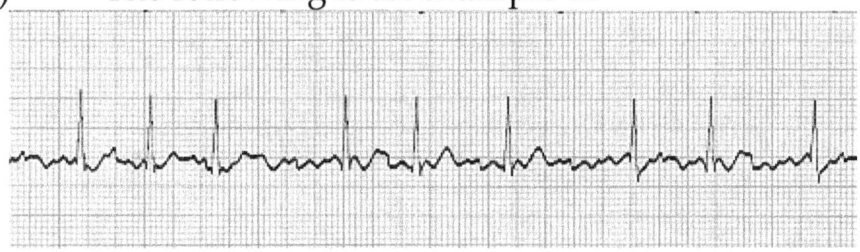
    a. Atrial fibrillation
    b. Ventricular fibrillation
    c. AV node fibrillation
    d. Stroke

33)   Which of the following is characterized by no identifiable P waves
    with fibrillatory F waves seen in all leads?
    a. Asystole
    b. Sinoatrial fibrillation
    c. Atrial fibrillation
    d. Ventricular fibrillation

34)   Which of the following is true about premature ventricular complexes?
    a. They do not show up on an EKG reading
    b. They arise from irritable sites in the atria
    c. The QRS complex is typically less than 0.12
    d. They may appear in the same shape or in different shapes

35)   Which of the following could cause a premature ventricular complex?
    a. Increased catecholamines
    b. Decreased blood pressure
    c. Increased ventricular activity
    d. Decreased heart rate

36) What is the term used for 3 or more PVC's in a row at a rate of over 100 BPM for more than 30 seconds?
a. Sinus tachycardia
b. Ventricular tachycardia
c. Sinoatrial bradycardia
d. None of the above

37) Which of the following is false about ventricular fibrillation?
a. It is not life threatening
b. It is caused by quivering of the ventricles
c. The rhythm is chaotic
d. It is characterized by waves that vary in shape and size

38) The following is an example of

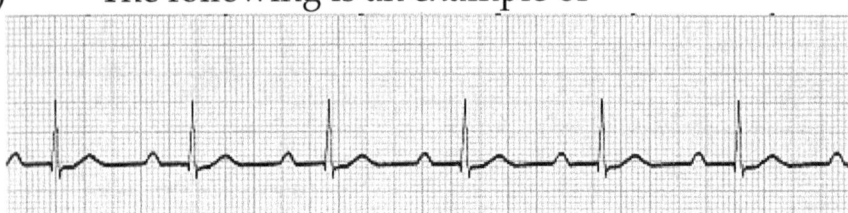

a. Asystole
b. First degree heart block type I
c. Normal sinus rhythm
d. Sinus bradycardia

39) The following is an example of

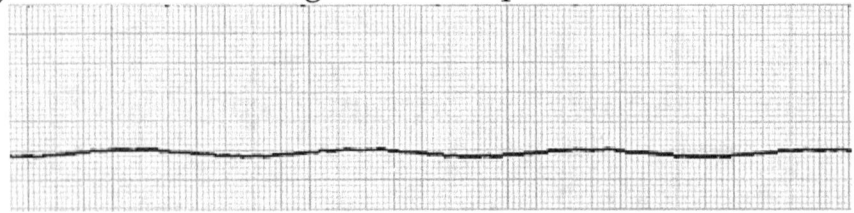

a. Asystole
b. First degree heart block type I
c. Normal sinus rhythm
d. Sinus bradycardia

40) Type II second degree AV block:
a. Conducted P waves are normal and PR intervals are normal
b. Conducted PR waves are normal with unreliable QRS intervals
c. Conducted P waves have constant PR interval, but there are non-conducted P waves

d. None of the above

Part One Answers

1) B
2) D
3) C
4) A
5) C
6) C
7) A
8) C
9) D
10)   D
11)   C
12)   B
13)   D
14)   C
15)   A
16)   B
17)   B
18)   A
19)   D
20)   C
21)   C
22)   B
23)   D
24)   D
25)   C
26)   A
27)   C
28)   B
29)   D
30)   B

31)	A
32)	A
33)	C
34)	D
35)	A
36)	B
37)	A
38)	B
39)	A
40)	C